WATER, VITAMINS, MINERALS

AND

DIETARY NEEDS

FOR

GOATS

A SIMPLE GUIDE

Felicity McCullough

Paperback Edition

My Lap Shop Publishers
Plymouth, England
www.mylapshop.com

ISBN: 978-1-78165-049-3

Series: Goat Knowledge 11

Table of Contents

Introduction

Please see disclaimer section

Page 57

Nutrition is fundamental to your business because it is the basis for production. When talking about nutrition, it is the nutrients and not the food or feed that is important. There is no single food that will meet all the goat's requirements.

In this guide we will first go over what nutrients are essential for goats and then we will discuss production requirements.

Essential Nutrients

There are six essential nutrients which will be discussed in this book. These are water, protein, carbohydrates, fat, vitamins and minerals.

A goat's nutritional requirements depend on a number of factors. These factors include species, sex, production cycle, location, level of production and weather.

Water

The Importance Of Water

Water is essential for life.

Animals and even humans can survive longer without food than without water. The body is predominantly water. Water is essential for a number of bodily functions.

How much water an animal needs depends on a variety of factors including species, climate and level of production. Milk is mostly water as well Does (female goats) that are lactating have the highest water requirements. You need to be concerned with both the quality and quantity of water.

Dry Matter (DM)

Pretty much everything that you can feed a goat has a certain amount of water. When formulating diets for goats, you need to keep this in mind because the diet is usually formulated on top of dry matter (DM).

Dry matter is what is left over after the water is removed. Lettuce, for instance, has 95% water and 5% of DM.

The more water that is contained in a feed, means that the animals will need to consume more of said feed, to achieve the required nutrient levels.

Keep in mind that just because there is water in pretty much every food that is given to goats, their requirements are so high that they need to always have fresh water available to them.

Protein

The two arguably most important nutrients in regards to the rumen health are protein and carbohydrates.

Protein is the most expensive ingredient. It is a source of energy as well. If you feed too much protein, it will be converted to fat.

Protein Sources

There are two major sources of protein. There is the protein that is broken down and used by the microbes in the rumen (a chamber of the stomach) and then there is the protein that gets to the abomasum (another chamber of the stomach). The latter protein is called bypass protein.

The microbes themselves often get to the abomasum as well and can be considered a source of bypass protein.

There are a number of ways that protein can be protected from digestion within the rumen.

As stated before, each feedstuff has all of the nutrients in differing amounts. In terms of protein, corn cobs and straw, grain and grass hay have relatively low levels of protein.

The two feedstuffs that have high levels are soybean meal at 49% and fish meal at 66%. The major problem with fish meal is that it can't be given to commercial milking goats, because it produces off flavours in the milk.

You can get high levels of protein in fresh-grown pasture and alfalfa hay depending on the level of growth.

Protein Versus Nitrogen

Protein and nitrogen have a relationship. Nitrogen is the basis for protein. This is why cattle are fed urea, which is basically non-protein nitrogen.

In charts, it is considered to have 288% protein levels. It can only be included as part of a ration.

The microbes in the rumen are able to convert the nitrogen into protein. This is why ruminants don't really require that high quality protein, except when you are talking about bypass protein.

It goes both ways though. Protein can be broken down and the nitrogen released. This is a problem when you over feed protein because there is too much nitrogen that can't be used. This unused nitrogen is then released into the environment, polluting it.

Protein Requirements

Protein requirements vary from animal to animal. Protein needs varies even within the same animal depending on a number of factors, including what the animal is producing.

Older animals need less protein than younger animals that are growing.

Protein requirements are usually measured with crude proteins, when you are balancing diets.

There are three types of protein: undegradable protein, metabolizable protein and degradable intake protein.

Undegradable protein is considered when balancing as percentage of bypass protein.

Metabolizable protein is both bypass protein and the protein provided from the microbes.

It isn't usually used to balance diets.

Degradable intake protein is the protein that the microbes get to and break down, within the rumen.

Carbohydrates

Energy is essential for all living things. We often refer to energy as carbohydrates or carbs.

Energy and protein need to be present in the rumen, because the microbes need both to make volatile fatty acids, which is what is actually absorbed from the rumen. This is the major source of energy for the ruminant.

Nutritional Requirements And Measurements

Energy is measured as calories. Calories are the building block of other nutrients. If there is too much energy in a diet, that energy is stored as fat.

It can also be measured as total digestible nutrients (TDN), metabolizable energy and net energy.

TDN is the crudest measurement. Goats and sheep use TDN usually.

Metabolizable energy and net energy are used for chickens and cows.

Sources Of Carbs

Cereal grains are high in energy as are oats and corn. Oats contain around 76% and corn 88%.

Forages such as silage, pasture and hay can have moderate amounts depending on when they were cut. Corn cobs and oat straw have low levels.

Fat

Fat is also a source of energy. In fact, fat provides more than two times more energy than both protein and carbohydrates.

Importance Of Fats

Usually fats are not considered when formulating a diet, even though there are a number of essential fatty acids that are required for health.

Fat is important because it provides heat, insulation and body protection.

Fats are used in the diet to manipulate the meat profile of the finished carcass.

Fat Requirements And Sources

Fat is the cheapest source of energy. Ruminants need only less than 4% in their diets.

Feeds that have high levels of fat include vegetable fat, whole soybeans and whole cottonseed.

Vegetable fat is liquid and usually mixed into feed to reduce dust and make the feed taste better. Whole soybeans have 18.8% fat and whole cottonseed has 17.8%.

Vitamins

There are two types of vitamins: water-soluble and fat-soluble.

Water-soluble vitamins include B and C.

Fat-soluble vitamins include A, D, E and K.

Vitamin Requirements And Function

Requirements increase with age and are responsible for a number of functions in the body.

Some vitamins are produced within the body while others need to come from the diet.

Vitamins are usually measured in international units and the general requirements are small yet essential.

There are a number of diseases that arise as a result of vitamin deficiencies.

Vitamin K and the B-complex vitamins are examples of vitamins that are produced in the body. They are manufactured by microbes in the rumen.

The B-complex vitamins can be supplemented in goats that have slow rumens, to try to stimulate them.

Vitamin A is manufactured from Beta Carotene. Beta Carotene can be found in green pasture, dehydrated forage and as a vitamin supplement.

Vitamin D is found in the sun, in hays and in vitamin supplements.

Vitamin E is found in legume hay, dehydrated alfalfa, wheat germ and vitamin supplements.

There are two types of vitamin K, K2 and K1. K2 can be produced in the rumen and K1 is found in leafy feedstuffs.

Minerals

Minerals are divided into macro-minerals and micro-minerals. Both are essential.

The difference is that animals require more of the macro-minerals than the micro-minerals to stay healthy. The levels needed are small for both.

Goats normally require grams of the macro-minerals and milligrams or less of the micro-minerals.

Mineral Functions And Requirements

Similar to vitamins, minerals have a variety of functions in the body and even though only small amounts are required, they are essential to health.

There are a number of diseases that can develop if the animal gets too little or too much of these minerals. This is why it is so important to consult your veterinarian about supplementation.

The most important mineral requirements include selenium, copper, calcium, phosphorus, sodium and chloride.

Different feeds have different levels of minerals. For example, bone meal and ground limestone are important for calcium.

Interactions Between Nutrients

In order to better understand nutrients and nutritional requirements, the nutrients are discussed separately and divided into sections. In truth, though, they are all mixed up in the feeds that we offer our goats. They are not isolated and they interact between and among themselves. This does have its effects.

For instance, calcium and phosphorus both interact. You need to keep feeds with a two to one ratio in terms of calcium to phosphorus.

The ratio is especially important for male goats, because if this proportion is off balance it can lead to the development of urinary stones.

Some other examples include copper and sulphur, vitamin E and selenium and even energy and protein. There are also a number of vitamin and mineral interactions.

Fibre

Fibre is not a nutrient in the traditional sense. Nevertheless, it is an essential component of the ruminant diet. Rumen health depends on the amount of fibre in the diet.

The type of volatile fatty acid that is produced in the rumen can be manipulated by the amount of fibre in the diet. Feed rich in fibre are converted to propionic acid by the microbes in the rumen.

The digestibility of the feed also depends on fibre; the more fibre, the less digestible the feed. It can be measured by two different methods: acid detergent fibre and neutral detergent fibre.

Requirements For Production

All living things have nutritional requirements. This has been studied for many, many years and a number of tables have been drawn up and revised.

There are a number of factors that interfere with nutritional requirements. This is covered more in depth in the guide entitled Managing Goat nutrition: What You Need To Know A Simple Guide.

Generally speaking, nutritional requirements will change depending on gender, species, and even production levels and stages of life.

Does that are dry and bucks out of breeding season only require maintenance levels of nutrition, which is the lowest requirements.

On the other hand, dairy does at the peak of lactation require the highest levels of nutrition.

The maintenance requirements for goats are higher than for sheep and dairy goats' nutrition requirements are higher than for meat and fibre goats.

Goats with the best mohair are usually raised in the areas with the worst nutrition.

Size In Weight Requirements

Goats, whose weight is high, have higher nutritional requirements, yet they need a lot more of a less nutrient-dense feed and less percentage of its body weight.

On the other hand, smaller animals eat less food, yet that feed needs to be denser with higher levels of protein, energy and digestibility.

Age On Requirements

Doelings tend to weigh less and eats less. They need a higher percentage of TDN, more digestible feed with higher levels of energy.

Younger animals require more calcium and phosphorus.

This is why doelings should be kept separate from adult does.

Adult females are bigger and they need to eat more of a less dense diet. They need to eat more pounds of dry matter, energy, protein and calcium and phosphorus.

Stage And Level Of Production

Generally speaking, as productivity increases, animals need more nutrients in more nutrient dense feeds.

Does in gestation need a more nutrient dense feed, especially later in gestation.

It is important to offer proper amounts and not to exaggerate, because a lot of the energy goes into the foetus growth and if the foetus grows too much it will cause problems at kidding.

The need for minerals goes up as gestation progresses, except for calcium which decreases in early lactation.

The need for protein jumps during lactation.

The need for calcium and phosphorus are highest during late gestation and lactation.

The more kids there are, the higher the need for dry matter, energy, protein, calcium and phosphorus. The doe that has more kids needs a more nutrient-dense diet.

The more milk produced, the higher the level of energy, protein and minerals needed.

Growth

Growing animals require more energy and protein levels. There is a bit of room to manoeuvre depending on your system.

There are ways to make kids grow faster or slower. Whether a kid is early maturing or late maturing depends on genetics.

Younger animals convert feed more efficiently yet need more protein. The decision to grow your kids fast or slow depends on what you feel is most economical for your particular farm.

Meat goats can gain about 100 grams per day. As they gain weight, they will need to eat more. The smaller they are, the more protein and the more concentrated the diet needs to be.

Gender

There are different genetic types. These include dairy, Boer and indigenous. Each type has their unique nutritional needs.

Boers need to eat more than dairy goats. Boers are more efficient in food conversion. Dairy goats need a more energy dense diet.

Weather

Animals in cold weather need more nutrients than animals that are located in warm weather.

Summary

Goats require six essential nutrients, water, protein, energy, fat, vitamins and minerals. The feed they eat usually contains more than one of these essential nutrients, and vary in combinations. Balancing what the animal's nutritional needs are very important and vary from species to species, at different ages and stages and level of production and can be influenced by the weather.

Change to diet needs to be gradual, whether an adult, or to a doeling. Smaller does doesn't need to eat as much, however the smaller doe still has the requirements for more nutrients.

A buck needs more dry matter and energy than a doe; however both require the same amount of protein. As does eat less they need a higher amount of protein in their diet. Feed males and females differently to meet their individual nutritional needs, both in terms of quantity and quality based on your need to meet the most economical performance gain.

Resources

Goat Lap Shop

www.goatlapshop.com

A Simple Guide To The Goat's Digestive System

Database of veterinarians

Diseases of Goats (article)

Golden Guernsey Goats

Goat Basics

Goat Videos

How To Keep Goats Healthy

Nigerian Dwarf Goats (article)

Nimbkar Boer Goat (article)

Schallenberg Virus (article)

Success Guide For Raising Healthy Goats

The Fun of Goats (article)

Copyright 2012

My Lap Shop Publishers

be   addressed   to:
My Lap Shop Publishers, 91
Mayflower Street, Unit 222,
Plymouth, Devon PL1 1SB UK

Publishers

My Lap Shop Publishers

91 Mayflower Street, Unit 222,

Plymouth, Devon, PL1 1SB

United Kingdom

Tel: +44 (0)871 560 5297

www.mylapshop.com

www.goatlapshop.com

First Edition September 2012

ISBN: - 978-1-78165-049-3

Acknowledgements

The publisher thanks Danielle Shurskis for her support and help in bringing these series of books to publication.

About Felicity McCullough

Felicity McCullough has written several books about preventative health care for goats. The website dedicated to goats www.goatlapshop.com has a wide variety of topics and resources that relate to goats, including other guides in the Goat Knowledge Series and the Charlie And Isabella's Magical Adventures Series of Children's Books, suitable for bed-time reading that are beautifully illustrated.

Goat Knowledge Series Titles

How To Keep Goats Healthy #1
ISBN: 978-1-78165-021-9
Golden Guernsey Goats #2
ISBN: 978-1-78165-022-6
A Simple Guide To The Goat's
Digestive System #3
ISBN: 978-1-78165-024-0
Success Guide For Raising
Healthy Goats #4
ISBN: 978-1-78165-026-4
Managing Goat Nutrition: What
You Need To Know A Simple
Guide #5
ISBN: 978-1-78165-027-1
Plants And Goats An Easy To
Read Guide #6
ISBN: 978-1-78165-038-7
Goat Housing, Bedding, Fencing,
Exercise Yards And Pasture
Management Guide #7
ISBN: 978-1-78165-040-0

Weaning Your Goat Kids A Simple Guide #8
ISBN: 978-1-78165-042-4
How To Breed Goats And Manage Gestation A Simple Guide #9
ISBN: 978-1-78165-045-5
Milking Your Goats What You Need To Know Guide #10
ISBN: 978-1-78165-047-9

Other Goat Books And Articles

by Felicity McCullough

www.goatlapshop.com

Boar Goats

Charlie And Isabella's Magical Adventure

Charlie And Isabella Meet Jacob

Charlie And Isabella's Second Adventure With Jacob

Charlie And Isabella's Magical Adventures Compendium

Diseases of Goats

Goat Basics

Goat Breed: Golden Guernsey Goats

Goat Videos

How To Keep Goats Healthy

Nigerian Dwarf Goats

Nimbkar Boer Goat

Raising Goats Easy Guide To Raising and Caring for Goats

The Fun of Goats

My Lap Shop Publishers

Plymouth, England

www.mylapshop.com

Disclaimer

This book is meant to be STRICTLY AN EDUCATIONAL AND INFORMATIONAL TOOL ONLY. The suggestions contained in this material might not be suitable for everyone. It is not intended to provide diagnosis or treatment. The author obtained the information from sources believed to be reliable and from personal experience. Although the best effort was made by the author, there are no guarantees as to the accuracy or completeness of the contents within this work.

The author does not guarantee the accuracy of any information or content in resources or websites listed or cited within this work. Additionally, the author, publisher and distributors never give medical, legal, accounting or any other type of professional advice. The reader must always seek those services from competent professionals that can review the particular circumstances. Mention of any product, brand or website is NOT an endorsement or recommendation of that product, service or usage.

The medical field is a very dynamic field that is constantly undergoing research, modifications and advancements and therefore information contained in this book should always be researched further and A VETERINARIAN OR OTHER SPECIALIST SHOULD BE CONSULTED where appropriate.

Any and all application of the information contained in this book is of the sole responsibility of the person performing said action. The author, publisher and distributors particularly disclaim any liability, loss, or risk taken by individuals who directly or indirectly act on the information herein. All readers must accept full responsibility for their use of this material.

My Lap Shop Publishers
Plymouth, England
www.mylapshop.com